PEDIATRIC DENTISTRY: BUILDING A NO-FEAR PRACTICE

PEDIATRIC DENTISTRY: BUILDING A NO-FEAR PRACTICE

✦

Introducing Children to a Lifetime of Positive Dental Care

Allan R. Pike, DDS, MS

iUniverse, Inc.

New York Lincoln Shanghai

PEDIATRIC DENTISTRY: BUILDING A NO-FEAR PRACTICE

Introducing Children to a Lifetime of Positive Dental Care

Copyright © 2006 by Allan R. Pike, DDS, MS

iUniverse books may be ordered through booksellers or by contacting:

iUniverse
2021 Pine Lake Road, Suite 100
Lincoln, NE 68512
www.iuniverse.com
1-800-Authors (1-800-288-4677)

ISBN-13: 978-0-595-39184-4 (pbk)
ISBN-13: 978-0-595-83574-4 (ebk)
ISBN-10: 0-595-39184-2 (pbk)
ISBN-10: 0-595-83574-0 (ebk)

Printed in the United States of America

To Marney, the love of my life for over 40 years, advisor, critic, and friend; and to our wonderful children, Michelle, Steven, and Jamie.

Contents

ACKNOWLEDGEMENTS

Thanks to my most capable and patient editor, Jill Kelly; to my parents and my brothers, Malcolm and Larry; and to all my office staff, friends, and teachers who have guided and inspired me over the years, including Leonard Boeder, Larry Turner, Rodney Dunn, Dean Nyquist, Donald Porter, Evelyn Strange, Duane Paulson, Walter Lindsay, J. Henry Clarke, Prashant Gagneja, Felix Loeb, and especially my Aunt Rose, who by her example showed me how to respect and love children.

1

CHILDREN DON'T FORGET

Psychologists tell us that a traumatic experience during childhood may affect the way we feel and behave later in life. Nowhere is this truer than with visits to the dentist. As an experienced pediatric dentist, I have observed many fearful children who have had painful dental experiences. These experiences often lead them to have dental anxiety and to avoid the dentist. Many of these children will carry these fears well into their adult lives.

We also know that parents who have had a traumatic experience at the dentist may, knowingly or unknowingly, transmit their anxiety to their children. The mother of one of my child patients told me this story:

I am 34 years old and still need to be constantly reminded and nagged to go to the dentist. Although my dentist now is sensitive to my needs, I still dread the experience. I attribute this to my childhood dental experience. I was apprehensive and was crying so they stuck blocks in my mouth to keep my mouth open. I remember the gagging sensation and the feeling of helplessness. I viewed going to the dentist as a penance for eating sweets…much like punishment. I felt ashamed of cavities. I've even experienced some apprehension in bringing my child to the dentist.

I hear stories like this more often than I like. While I can't vouch for their accuracy, the bottom line is that this is how these adults remember their childhood trips to the dentist. These visits clearly made lasting and damaging impressions.

When I was 3, they put me in a big chair, strapped my wrists down, and numbed my mouth with a huge needle. I cried and was told to stop being a baby and stop crying NOW or else! When they started drilling, it still hurt. I kicked my feet, which they then strapped down. I was crying and screaming. My mom took a picture of me after the teeth caps were done. I was lying on the floor at our house with my blanket. That picture breaks my heart even today. I hated the dentist from then on. It's been 32 years. My anxiety follows me as an adult with two children. I haven't been in a dentist chair for 10 years! The fear sticks with you.

◆   ◆   ◆

When I was 4 years old, I went to the dentist. My mom was in the waiting room. They poked me so many times my gums were bleeding. I was screaming! They wouldn't let my mom in to see me. My mother bombarded the receptionist to get me out of there. I have not been to the dentist for 15 years! To this day I get panic attacks when I have a shot.

◆   ◆   ◆

When I was 3, I didn't cooperate very well, so with my father's help, they strapped me down. It's been 33 years and I still remember the utter panic I experienced. I still struggle with claustrophobia.

◆   ◆   ◆

At the age of 4, I visited the dentist and, unfortunately I wished for many years that I had not. This visit is one of my earliest and most vivid—sitting in a chair with my hands tied to the sides of the chair and a big black padded bar across my lap. I don't remember crying or "being naughty," just afraid. It has been 36 years and I still get very anxious when visiting the dentist.

◆   ◆   ◆

Between the ages of 6 and 10, I saw a dentist who drilled on my teeth without the aid of Novocain. He had straps for your legs and arms and said that I should try to "breathe away the pain." Needless to say I was petrified and it hurt. When I objected, he told me I was not being "good." My mother was never allowed back in the examination room with me. When I complained to her, she was unsympathetic and said I was a sissy. It has been hard to trust anyone in the dental profession. Last year I finally got the courage to make an appointment.

◆   ◆   ◆

When my grandson Michael was 3, he was taken to a dentist who would not allow his mom to be with him. This dentist strapped him down and paid no attention to his fears and treated him rudely and roughly. Before this experience, he enjoyed having his teeth brushed. He was, by nature, a happy and compliant child. After the experience, he had to be held down while having his teeth brushed. He would scream hysterically and he even vomited several times. His mother has learned much about child psychology, parenting, and respecting the thoughts and words of children since then and would never allow this to happen now. But to this day Michael is like stone when he has to see the dentist, which is something he does ONLY when he has no choice.

Stories like these do not appear to be isolated cases. Researchers have studied the long-term effects of forceful methods on dental attitudes. In one study, professional interviewers spoke to 1000 adults selected at random in Seattle, Washington[1]. Of these adults, 204 said they were highly fearful of the dentist. Of these 204 fearful people, 66% reported

---

1.   Milgrom P, Fiset L, *et al.* The prevalence and practice management consequences of dental fear in a major U.S. city. *JADA* 1988;116:641-647.

that they had acquired that fear in early childhood. That means of 1000 adults, 150 (15%) are highly fearful because of a bad childhood dental experience. Extending this into the general population means that at least 30 million Americans are afraid to go to the dentist because of a bad childhood experience. A 1984 study had similar results: Of 160 dental phobics, 85% of them related their fear to a bad childhood dental experience[2]. Additionally, a 1991 study showed that of 80 dental phobics, 70% attributed their fears to childhood experience[3].

Because dental phobics avoid going to the dentist, early diagnosis and early simple, inexpensive, and painless treatment is impossible. If they are lucky, the tooth can be salvaged with root canal therapy and a crown. When it is too late for that or they can't afford it, the tooth gets extracted. Eventually as this scenario repeats itself, bridgework or dentures become necessary, all because of a bad experience as a child getting a primary tooth repaired. What a terrible price to pay!

And, as we know, it is not just the ability to chew and the health of the jaw that is lost. Appearance, self-confidence, and subsequent treatment by teachers, supervisors, and friends are all affected by the state of the teeth. Chronic untreated gum disease is also one of the leading causes of bad breath, which has its own major social implications.

And of course, research now links low-grade chronic inflammation, which is common with untreated gum disease, with cardiovascular disease, while abscessed teeth can have life-threatening consequences, especially if the person is predisposed to heart valve or kidney problems. Joint replacement and stroke-prone people are also at risk from abscessed teeth. While such issues are not usually problems for chil-

---

2.   Berggren U, Meynert G. Dental fear and avoidance: Causes, symptoms, and consequences. *JADA* 1984; 109(2):247-251.

3.   Moore R, Brodsgaard I, Birn H. Manifestations, acquisition and diagnostic categories of dental fear in a self-referred population. *Behavior Res Ther* 1991;29(1):51-60.

dren, they are for adults with dental phobias based in traumatic childhood experiences.

After practicing pediatric dentistry with traditional methods of managing children for nearly 20 years, methods that made me uncomfortable and many of my child patients miserable, I knew I had to find a different way. This book describes the change I made by putting the child before the tooth. It is my goal to work towards eliminating traumatic experiences in the dental office so that all children grow up feeling good about going to the dentist.

2

MY STORY

I have been a practicing pediatric dentist for almost 40 years. For about half of that time, I used the traditional methods to get my work done, including all the classic behavior management techniques that would help me be efficient: tell-show-do, voice control, sedation, physical restraints, hand-over-mouth, and quiet rooms when necessary.

In the early years of my practice, when a child would "misbehave," I would wrap them up in a restraint and tough it out. I was always careful not to hurt them and I always gave an anesthetic, but sometimes they cried for the whole appointment. In retrospect, I never really knew for sure whether they were just scared or if the anesthetic didn't work.

Rather than "give in" to the child, I assumed the responsibility of getting the child's teeth restored no matter what. In addition, I assumed the responsibility of being the parent while the child was in my office. In fact, if the parent had done a poor job of teaching the child to behave and mind adults, I thought it was my job to correct that deficiency by whatever means necessary, so I could get the treatment done. In the end, I was exhausted, my assistant was drained, the parent rarely appreciated my effort, and the child, needless to say, was very unhappy.

And how do you think I acted when the next patient came in a few minutes later? I was still trembling from the last one, and my patience had already worn thin.

When the crying child had left, I used to rationalize away my feelings of distress. What a spoiled brat! Why weren't his parents teaching him to be mindful of adults? Besides, it couldn't have hurt—I gave him an anesthetic. Well, even it if did hurt a little, he'll forget it. Sadly I know now that this is not true. The children didn't forget and neither did I.

In the beginning, I hated doing things that way, but as the years went by, I got accustomed to the crying. I never liked it, but I thought it was simply something that I couldn't avoid. I had to get the job done and to teach the child that I was in charge and they'd better get used to it.

Unfortunately, what they really learned was to avoid the dentist whenever possible. When it was time for their six-month checkup, I noticed that some didn't want to come back. Big surprise! I remember a few times having to go out to the parking lot and help their mothers pull them out of the car. They usually had to go straight back into the crying room. It's sad for me to admit that I thought all this was necessary. Sadder still to admit that it took me almost two decades to change those methods.

While the behavior management methods that are taught and accepted do work, some of them achieve results at a high cost: instilling a long-term fear of the dentist. Even though many of us are reluctant to perform the more aggressive methods, as I was, we may view them as necessary in order to get the job done, as I used to.

We may well be under pressure from the parent to complete a procedure. The child may have been up during the night with a toothache, or the parent may have taken time off work to bring their child to you, or they may have driven a long distance and don't want to make two trips. It is very often the parent's expectation that we are going to fix their problem and do it today. When a child is resistant or scared or terrified or spoiled or obnoxious or unruly or cranky, there may be a number of pressing reasons to get the procedure done now and get it over with.

In private practice, there are also financial pressures. We are paid only for the work we do. Insurance plans do not have a billing code for coaxing. If nothing gets done, the overhead goes on but the income has stopped.

For the first two decades, I myself sometimes succumbed to these pressures. I felt that if I let a child get away without doing any treatment, he would not only get spoiled, but he would likely try the same tactic the next time. I was convinced that kids needed to learn who was in charge.

Looking for a better solution, I made an extensive study of tranquilizers and sedatives, but as I tried them, they only seemed to work about half the time. When they didn't work, the child had to go back into the crying room. I continued to look for the perfect drug, one that would always work. I never did find it. I did notice that if I increased the dose, the success rate went up; that is, the child was heavily sedated and I could do the treatment. However, some of those kids were pretty hard to wake up. That made me uneasy. Even with a reversal drug, I felt uncomfortable. Light sedation didn't work that well and heavy sedation had a potential for serious danger. There had to be a better way.

Occasionally I'd see a study in a dental journal about the long-term effects on children who had had a bad experience with a dentist. Data was beginning to accumulate that frightening childhood experiences were not soon forgotten. As adults, these people often avoided going to a dentist for routine care, which resulted in many of their teeth becoming so badly decayed that they had to be removed. I simply had to find a way to have children leave my office with a good memory of their visit.

Then it hit me. All I had to do was to decide in my own mind that the child's memory was more important than fixing the tooth. I really didn't need to worry about spoiling the child; that's a parenting issue. My job was to repair teeth in a way that made a child feel safe, comfortable, and not afraid to come back. That's when my approach to children began to change. I got rid of my restraining board and took the door off the quiet room. My focus shifted from relationships based on authority to pleasant memories and trust. With many years behind me now of this different approach, I believe that it is never necessary to use fear-producing methods of behavior management. There are always better alternatives.

This book describes some of these gentler, non-threatening methods for effective dental treatment of children. It is my experience that parents want dentists who will treat their children in a manner that is in the best long-term interest of their child, rather than a quick fix and a potentially damaging memory.

3

A BRIEF HISTORY OF BEHAVIOR MANAGEMENT IN THE DENTAL OFFICE

The more aggressive methods of restraint and management of children grew out of a different kind of dentistry and different attitudes about young people. To understand how managing children's behavior evolved, it may be helpful to look at some of the technical and cultural circumstances that existed in the past.

Emergency-Based Dentistry

Before 1900, little dental prevention was practiced; instead, dentistry was emergency-based. People waited until they had a painful problem before going to the dentist. The most common condition that dentists treated was the abscessed tooth, which usually came with infection, fever, pain, and swelling. In those pre-antibiotic years, a dental infection could be life threatening. It could spread unchecked, so it was important to deal with the tooth as quickly as possible.

It was also common in those days for patients to delay treatment until the pain and swelling were unbearable, most often because the treatment itself was associated with excruciating pain. By the time he reached a dentist, the patient was not in good spirits. Sleep had been lost. Eating had become difficult, if not impossible. Morale was low, and decision-making clouded. When distraught or terrified patients were not willing, they had to be restrained by whatever means necessary, and the tooth was extracted. Teeth and jawbones were commonly broken during the effort to remove the diseased tooth, and death frequently followed a few days later. According to public records called the "Bills of Mortality," for example, during a one-week period in 1623 in London, England, dental infections were the fifth leading cause of death[1]. It probably would not have occurred to the dentist to consider how the patient felt about treatment or its long-term psychological consequences.

There was little dental training, except apprenticeships, and physicians, barbers, and even blacksmiths did extractions. Laudanum, a mixture of opium and wine, did little to help the pain. General anesthesia was not developed until 1844, and local anesthesia not until 40 years after that. Even then, such anesthesia was not always safely applied, and it was only available in larger Eastern cities[1]. Most patients, sadly, had to simply "tough it out."

Cultural Attitudes about Children and Psychology

The relationship between children and authority figures and the development of the field of child psychology are other factors that enter into the picture. Over the last 100 years, there have been significant changes in both. In the late 19th century, corporal punishment was a commonly accepted practice in homes and schools. The saying "Spare the rod and spoil the child" was common. No one wanted a spoiled child so parents, teachers, clergymen, and doctors freely administered corporal punishment whenever they felt it was needed. The level of aggressive punishment that a society finds acceptable is important in understanding how methods of behavior management evolved in pediatric dentistry. If aggressive punishment was acceptable by parents, teachers, and clergy, it was equally acceptable by the child's dentist.

Coming as it did out of both emergency-based dentistry and corporal punishment as common circumstances, it is not surprising that methods of controlling children in dentistry evolved as they did.

---

1.   Clarke JH. Toothaches and death. *J History Dentistry* 1999;47:11-13.

Today, most of Western society has moved away from severe and aggressive discipline for children. But in the early part of the 20th century, child psychology was just beginning to emerge as a field of study, and scientists were just beginning to formally study the complexity of behavior and emotions. The medical profession, led by Freud, was also only beginning to realize that traumatic experiences during childhood could have profound effects later in life.

The acceptance of these new attitudes into dentistry was slow in coming. In 1939, for example, a highly respected pediatric dentist, M. Evangeline Jordan, DDS, had this to say about the "management of children who cry and struggle"[2]:

If a normal child will not listen but continues to cry and struggle, the following plan has never failed: explain to the parents that you will hold him until he stops crying, and dismiss them to the waiting room. With the right hand, hold a folded napkin over the child's mouth so arranged that it does not cover his nose, place the left arm around his head, and with the left hand gently but firmly hold his mouth shut…there will be little sound, and he will soon begin to reason. Have the nurse hold his hands and feet…

Many cases do require from a quarter to a half-hour to calm down, before you can finally remove the napkin.

If you give up without doing any work, the child has won the victory and you can never succeed with him. The worst feature of your not having been able to convince him that the work will not hurt lies in his impression of having won in a victorious struggle. This will make it doubly hard for the next dentist; or perhaps the disheartened parents will give up; then the subsequent ill health of the child should justly be laid at your door.

A few years later, in 1945, another respected teacher and director of the Department of Pediatric Dentistry at the University of Detroit, Walter C. McBride, DDS, wrote this about "incorrigible" children[3]:

2. Jordan ME. *Operative Dentistry for Children.* Brooklyn, NY: Dental Items of Interest Publishing Co., 1939; 9-10.
3. McBride WC. *Juvenile Dentistry.* 4th ed. Philadelphia, PA: Lea & Febiger, 1945; 43.

At times, in his practice, the author has resorted to the towel procedure to break down the iron will of an incorrigible patient. It is drastic, but "the spirit must be conquered before the flesh can be subdued." It may sound severe and unfair, but it is a measure of last resort and need be used but infrequently. With this type of patient, the mother must necessarily be excused and, as she leaves the room, the simple suggestion is made that the latch be turned on the door—otherwise, she will be back at the crucial moment and destroy all that has been accomplished.

McBride then goes on to describe a variation of Jordan's napkin method. He adds one important component: pinching the nose of the child shut and cutting off the air supply!

These behavior management techniques were effective—and efficient—but they did the job at the cost of a lifelong fear of the dentist. And even though they are on the decline, these methods do persist today. In 2002, a commonly used dental textbook *Dentistry for the Child and Adolescent*[4] included this passage:

The behavior modification method of aversive conditioning is also known as Hand-Over-Mouth Exercise, or by the acronym HOME. Its purpose is to gain the attention of a highly oppositional child so that communication can be established and cooperation obtained for a safe course of treatment. The technique fits the rules of learning theory: Maladaptive acts (screaming, kicking) are linked to restraint, and cooperative behavior is related to removal of the restriction (hand over mouth) and the use of positive reinforcement (praise). It is important to stress that aversive conditioning is not used routinely but as a method of last resort, usually with children 3 to 6 years of age having appropriate communicative abilities.

I too was taught this as a last-resort technique. Now I know that it and other aggressive methods are not necessary—ever. Furthermore, when a child is being physically restrained while having dental work done, how do we know for sure that it isn't hurting? All we know is that we gave an anesthetic. But in some cases, anesthetic doesn't work,

---

4.   McDonald RE. *Dentistry for Children and Adolescents*. 8th ed. St Louis, MO: Mosby Inc., 2004; 46.

due to infection or unusual body chemistry or anatomy. If an adult tells us that the shot didn't work, we give another injection or switch to another method or another type of anesthetic. But when a child says it still hurts, we may think the child is just scared and trying to get out of something. We need to trust children when they say, "Stop! You're hurting me!"

In addition, imagine how devastating it is when a parent or other adult-in-charge helps to hold the child down and becomes the source of pain and anxiety rather than being the one who protects from it. Such disappointment is why bad dental experiences are remembered so vividly for so many years.

Today most children who see a dentist do not face life-threatening complications. And our attitudes about children and their role in the family and in society have changed drastically. I believe it is time for us to let go of all outdated and aggressive ways of handling the children we see.

4

CURRENT METHODS OF TREATING UNWILLING CHILDREN

Some children are shy. It may be an inherited aspect of their personality or it may be learned. These shy children are very cautious about new things, new places, and new people. When a shy child meets a busy dentist, there can be a conflict. The child needs extra time, but the dentist doesn't have any.

Dental textbooks and training explain how to overcome that shyness by teaching us how to develop a relationship with the child. Before any dental work is done, we describe the procedure to the child using age-appropriate language and we give demonstrations. For many children, that's all there is to it and everything goes well. But for roughly one in five children, it's not enough. In spite of everything that we—and the parent—may do or say, the child remains cautious and fearful and does not allow treatment.

At this critical moment, if we use force, the child's shyness can transform into overt anxiety and resistance. This is the moment of choice for the dentist. Do we put the work and the tooth first or the child and his memories?

Dental schools train us for these situations with a variety of techniques. Here's a quick review of them and how they can sometimes lead to problems.

Voice Control

If gently explaining ahead of time what is to be done and giving a brief demonstration does not work and the child is still afraid, most of us are taught to move to "voice control." Our facial expression, tone, and volume gradually escalate to imply impending serious consequences. For example, we say softly, "Open, please." If nothing happens, we say, a little louder this time, "Bobby, please open your mouth." Again if nothing happens, our voice becomes loud and firm: "Bobby, open your mouth right now!" Bobby opens his mouth. Score: Dentist–1. Bobby–0.

But what about the next dental appointment? We think Bobby has learned to open his mouth when told to do so. But we know from surveys and professional experience that what Bobby has really learned is that the dentist has little regard for his fears and cannot be trusted to always be kind and gentle. This lesson is not soon forgotten.

Furthermore, even though the dentist using voice control is supposed to be putting on an act, it can occasionally go from just a show to real anger. At that point, the frustrated dentist is out of control and has crossed the line. Sometimes a dentist's patience can wear thin, and gentle suggestions can escalate to shouting, especially if it is late in the day and the previous patients were also uncooperative.

Hand Over Mouth Exercise (HOME)

Properly administered, HOME is done while the dentist is totally calm and in control. The dentist's hand is softly but firmly placed over the screaming child's mouth while the dentist calmly explains to the child that as soon as the noise stops, the hand will be removed. The danger with HOME is that the edge of the hand is very close to the child's nose and in the course of restraining a struggling child, the hand may inadvertently cover the nose, thus unintentionally cutting off all air. Furthermore, if the nose is congested because of a cold or allergy or, most likely, crying, breathing is further compromised. At the same time, psychiatrists tell us there is a definite correlation between a history of suffocation and breathing disorders such as hyperventilation, panic attacks, and even perhaps some forms of asthma[1]. The memory of being smothered is not soon forgotten.

Most parents will not allow HOME to be used on their child, and it has caused so much legal and public opinion trouble that its use is, fortunately, beginning to decline. In fact, HOME is prohibited by law in some states. In 1980, HOME was used by 90 % of practicing pediatric dentists where as in 2003 the number had declined to about 21%[2]. However, the technique is still taught in 15 of 54 American dental residency programs[3]. I would argue that it should not be taught or used at all.

Immobilization and Sedation

Immobilization and sedation are used rather widely by many dentists to facilitate completion of dental work when a child is unable or unwilling to sit still. According to a 2003 survey of pediatric dentists, nearly 70% said they used immobilization with non-sedated children regularly. About 50% used sedation and immobilization simultaneously[4].

Yet let's look at what happens when a child is immobilized. If a thrashing, terrified child is forcibly wrapped up in a restraining device, all dignity, self-control, and self-esteem is lost. If the child is struggling, the tendency is for the dentist to adjust the fasteners of the restraining device a little tighter. But if it's too tight, it can inhibit the normal chest expansion associated with breathing. The device must be loose enough to allow relaxed breathing.

1. Bouwer C, Stein DJ. Association of panic disorder with a history of traumatic suffocation. *Am J Psychiatry* 1997 Nov;154:1566-1570.
2. Adair SM, *et al*. Survey of members of American Academy of Pediatric Dentists on their use of behavior management techniques. *Pediatric Dentistry* 2004;26(2):159-166.
3. Adair SM, *et al*. Survey of behavior management teaching in pediatric dentistry advanced education programs. *Pediatric Dentistry* 2004;26(2):151-158.
4. Adair SM, *et al*. Survey of members.

Having the dental assistant or parent hold the child's arms and legs from moving usually does not restrict chest movements, so it can be safer on a sedated child. The downside, however, is that if a parent is restraining a child who is too lightly sedated or not sedated at all, it can permanently harm the child. The parent's normal role is to protect. If a child experiences the parent as not protecting but instead as acting as an accomplice, it can be devastating. I have more than once seen a child denounce the parent and refuse to talk or touch them after such an experience. It is not soon forgotten. Here's the viewpoint of a woman in her 30s:

"Can you imagine a mother siding with the dentist and helping him hold me down while he fixed my teeth? I remember my mother looking down at me not the least bit sorry and telling me I'd get over it. I'll never forgive her for that."

Yes, immobilization expedites treatment. Yes, the parent won't have to make another trip to the dentist and lose more time from work. And yes, the dentist will not have wasted valuable time. But at what price? It is likely that the child will, at some conscious or unconscious level, remember the event for many years.

And even though the dentist's intentions are good, the end result is that the child feels violated and tortured. Children think in the "now," not in the future. They don't understand that a small cavity left unfilled can later become a big one and that eventually the tooth will abscess and cause them much pain. What they will remember is that *"the mean dentist yelled at me and wouldn't let me go and poked a big needle in my mouth. I'm never going back there again."*

On the other hand, if the child is given a sedative, and it works, which for me was about half the time, the immobilizing device keeps the calmed, sleepy child contained. But what happens when sedation doesn't work? Any given drug does not affect all people in the same way. Some children need more (or less) sedative to achieve ideal sedation. If a child overreacts to the normal dose of a sedative, he not only falls asleep but he is also hard to wake up. His breathing slows and his blood pressure drops.

There are reversal drugs, but many dentists become a little unnerved using strong sedatives, fearing some permanent consequence. So the tendency is to play it safe and dose on the light side. While this is safer, it increases the chances of the child being under-dosed, which can lead, paradoxically, to hyperactivity rather than sedation. When this happens, the best thing to do is send the child home and try again another day with a different dose. But that's not what usually happens.

In the real world, the expectations of both the parent and the dentist are that something is going to get done today. We drove all the way over here. I took time off work. A drug's been given. Let's just get it done once and for all. Besides, the child is all wrapped up and can't move, and he'll probably forget the incident in a day or two. While this may make sense, in reality there is a chance that another dental phobic will be created.

Is it ever okay to hold a child down in order to complete a dental treatment? Certainly, if the child's life is at risk, such action can be rationalized. If a child has an abscessed tooth and there is a clear and likely possibility that the associated swelling and infection could endanger his life and no other gentler course of action is possible, then immobilizing may be justified. But to do so for convenience or in anticipation of some future problem does not justify the potential damage done to the child's psyche and self-esteem. In fact, long-term bad effects happen often enough so as not to justify the use of force in all but the rarest of instances. In most cases, infection can be treated medically first, then surgically in a few weeks when the urgency is gone.

5

WHY SOME DENTISTS USE THESE TECHNIQUES

The behavior management techniques described in Chapter 4 are very efficient. However, many children who receive this type of treatment develop a fear of going to the dentist. So why do we continue to use them?

First, these techniques have been legitimized as accepted practices. They are taught in our dental textbooks and our dental school classes, making them seem acceptable to—and promoted by—the profession. At the same time, sensitivity to the potential for dental anxiety is not always a part of our standard training.

Secondly, these techniques work. Dentists who use them are able to treat unwilling patients. This saves the parent additional visits and money while making the most economical use of the dentist's time and facilities.

The Task Completion Syndrome

We dentists take pride in our work. Getting a procedure done on time and doing a good job are basic elements of our dental education. When I was in dental school, the issues of time and quality were emphasized. We had a limited amount of time to produce a high-quality product. Given an *unlimited* amount of time, most of my classmates could produce a beautiful, well-fitting crown, for example. But those of us who could do it well—and fast—rose to the top of the class. Similarly, if I did something well but never got it finished, I got no credit at all. So starting on time and finishing on time were often a measure of success.

For most of us, the concept of finishing things starts long before dental school. From early childhood, our culture places emphasis on task completion, which is rewarded with praise and good grades. Later, as an adult, task completion is directly linked to salary and advancement, markers of professional success. Hence, when a dentist starts to prep a tooth, he has an overwhelming urge to complete the job, even over the objections of the child. He may well see stopping in the middle of the task as a failure rather than good judgment.

For example: You're restoring a tooth on a 5-year-old. Everything is going fine—your quality is excellent and you've got 15 minutes before your next patient. Suddenly, for no apparent reason, the child begins to fidget and object.

You tell him quietly, "Hold still so I can do a good job." He does so for about 10 seconds and then begins to whimper.

"Just hang on," you say a little louder, "we'll be done in two minutes."

His whimpers escalate to crying, and then he's making efforts to sit up. Getting a little stressed and impatient, you blurt out, "Be quiet and hold still!" This has no effect.

Now you're working as fast as you can, but things are getting out of control. Your left arm, which a few minutes ago was gently cradling his head, now tightens to hold it still. Your assistant stops suctioning and holds his hands so he won't grab yours. Your pace becomes feverish. The child is screaming now, and your arm is starting to ache and your assistant is having a hard time holding him down. "Just another few seconds and we'll be done," you say, all but shouting. "There! It's done!"

You're all exhausted. Hoping to turn a bad situation around, you say to the child, "Now, that wasn't really so bad, was it?"

He's still crying and yells out, "I don't like you!"

You try to compose yourself, and as you go into the break room, the assistant takes the child out to his mother. Seeing her child distraught, she asks, "What happened?"

"Oh," remarks your assistant as you've trained her to say, "he got a little tired at the end, but he'll be okay in a few minutes."

This scenario is so common that for many dentists, it is all in a day's work. It comes with the territory. Out of self-preservation, we become numb to the child's discomfort because we and the parent—and our culture—have placed too much emphasis on task completion. The task has become more important than the child's memory of the event.

A Sense of Urgency: Medical Concerns

Most of us are familiar with the medical term "urgent care." If we experience a life-threatening condition like a heart attack, stroke, burn, or car accident, we go to an urgent care clinic or an emergency room for immediate help. In dentistry, we rarely see life-threatening conditions anymore, so we are seldom required to do anything immediately to save a life.

However, dentists are trained to be concerned about the possibility of the spread of a dental infection. Some take this to mean that they should take action whenever possible, including the immediate extraction of an offending tooth. Unfortunately for the child patient, it is often difficult to completely numb an abscessed tooth as the infection interferes with the chemistry of the local anesthetic. Faced with the potential spread of infection, a dentist may choose to remove the tooth now even if it means that a "little" pain must be endured.

The dentist then gives the anesthetic, waits 10 minutes, and begins taking out the tooth, but as the tooth is being loosened, the child may show signs of pain. However, the decision has already been made to remove the tooth today: the anesthetic has been given, the forceps are already on the tooth. It is very easy now for the dentist to ignore the child's protests and stay the course. With a quick twist of the wrist and a scream, it is out! "Thank goodness that's over and we're done," think the parent and the dentist.

But that's not what the child thinks. The child thinks, "I don't like going to the dentist. Can I trust my parent? I'm certainly never going to come here anymore." And in many cases, another course of action was possible that would have saved the child's feelings and his long-term dental health.

A Sense of Urgency: Parental Pressure

A second sense of urgency can be created by parental pressure. Frequently a dentist is pressured by a parent to get something done at that moment, whether the child is willing or not. As we've seen, the parent may well have good reasons: "I don't want my child to miss any more school" or even "The traffic driving over here is awful and stressful. I don't want to make another trip."

Sometimes they don't understand the potential long-term consequences; they don't think about how the child will feel about today's dental visit in 6 months or 20 years. They're thinking, "I haven't got time for another visit."

And occasionally they are even insensitive to their child's feelings: "He's a wimp; let's just get it done" or "If we don't hurry up and get this done, my two other kids will miss their ball game."

In most of these cases, the dentist may feel pressured to please the parent—who's paying the bill—rather than safeguard the feelings and memories of the child.

Enough Is Enough! The Exasperation Factor

Some children can try our patience. We do everything right and still they refuse to let us fix their teeth. We're patient, we carefully explain everything in advance, we use age-appropriate language. We let them watch other visibly relaxed children having their dental work done. We have a rehearsal visit to practice the sights and sounds of dental instruments, and still they won't let us do anything. Some are simply born cautious and shy. Many times early in my career, I had the urge to just hold them still and get the job done. In some cases, I actually did just that.

The parents of these children can also be just as frustrated. They often asked me to just go ahead and do something. "Let's just do it and get it over with!" they'd say. "Besides, in a few minutes he'll get over it." Sometimes in the past I complied with their wishes.

Now I don't think that way anymore.

Cultural Issues: The Parent's Role

Views on how children should be raised vary widely in the United States. Some parents tend to be more permissive, while others lean more toward seeing themselves as authority figures who are in total control.

While I do think that small children need to mind their parents and other adults, I don't think the dental office is the place to learn this lesson. The dentist is not the parent, nor should the dentist compensate for a parent's inability to parent. It's the parent's role, not the dentist's, to teach the child life's lessons. Such teaching should start at home, long before the child's first dental visit.

Cultural Issues: The Dentist's Role

In the past, when a child in school got out of line, the teacher or principal became the disciplining parent. If discipline was needed, physical punishment was administered on the spot, so it is understandable that such an attitude would carry over to the dental office and to another authority figure, the dentist. Furthermore, the dentist is a professional who knows what is best and who is in charge. Therefore, a firm hand with the child is considered necessary by many parents and dentists.

This is reflected in dental training. Dental schools are charged with training bright, scientifically minded people to be dentists. The pediatric dentist is taught in school to assume the responsibility for getting something done one way or another. My teachers used to tell me that I was the last resort. Often the child had already been to several other dentists and nothing could be done because of "bad behavior." If I did not do it, who would? Besides, as we've seen, most of the aggressive techniques have, for many years, been a part of formal dental education. That in itself sanctions and perpetuates these techniques, so it is no surprise that 92% of dentists surveyed still use voice control, 70% still use immobilization, and 20% still use hand-over-mouth[1].

In addition, customs and treatment methods in all professions are slow to change. We do things in a certain way because we have always done them that way. They seem to work, so why change? Thus, in spite of published studies that demonstrate and explain the potential long-term ill effects of aversive and forceful methods, they still continue to be commonly used.

The Financial Angle

There is an additional important reason why I used to use forceful methods: I did it to earn a living. If I were a teacher or psychotherapist, I would get paid for my appointments simply if the patient showed up. But as a dentist, I only get paid for what I accomplish, not for my time. If I allocated one hour of my time, for example, for a given child and got nothing done, I didn't get paid. I'd spent an hour coaxing, sweet-talking, pleading, and maybe even bribing the child yet had nothing to show for it financially. However, my office overhead was still there; the assistant, the rent, the utilities, and the equipment lease still needed to be paid. There was a good reason why I needed to get things done, regardless of whether the child objected. Like most dentists, I wasn't greedy. I worked hard and wanted to at least cover the overhead.

A Word about General Anesthesia and Hospital Use

Most parents readily agree to general anesthesia for their children when it seems warranted. But when they find out how much it is going to

---

1.   Adair SM, *et al.* Survey of members. 2004.

cost, many simply can't or won't afford it. Even with insurance, their out-of-pocket cost can often be more than $3,000 (as of 2006) and that does not include the dental work. Because they can't afford it, some families pressure the pediatric dentist to try sedation and to do the treatment in the office using local anesthetic but sedation doesn't always work. And, as you can already guess, when you combine a young child with many teeth needing extensive repair in the office under local anesthesia, you have a recipe for creating a lifelong dental phobic.

6

A GENTLER APPROACH: EMPOWERMENT AND CONTROL OF PAIN

As you can see, there are lots of good reasons why dentists—I among them—have felt that we needed to get something done even if the child was not happy about us doing it. However, if I had known then what I know now, I would have stopped using those forceful methods much sooner. It took many years before I recognized the long-term consequences of what I was doing and that it had to stop.

A Pivotal Decision

Since we now know that early childhood experiences are not soon forgotten and that most dental conditions are not life threatening, it is hard to justify the use of forceful methods to treat children's dental problems.

Parents breathe a sigh of relief when I tell them that it's essential that their child's visits to the dentist are associated with good memories and that I plan to do whatever is necessary to make sure their child leaves with a good memory. And I keep my word. And while we may agree, the parent and I, that a variety of behavior management methods for repairing a tooth are possible, it is always clear from the outset that if nothing works, force is not an option. (See Appendix I for a sample introductory letter that we send to the parents of new patients.)

Behind the gentler methods that I advocate are two basic principles. The first is to allow the child to have a sense of power or control. The second is to not hurt the child.

Control or Veto Power

Freedom, or self-control, is an instinctive need common to all of us. Young or old, rich or poor, we all want to feel in control of our lives. It is a hard-wired trait, which probably evolved because it favored survival. Dentists can capitalize on that instinct by giving children a feeling of control.

To feel safe at the dentist's office, the child must have veto power. He must know that when he says, "Stop," the dentist or hygienist will stop, even when they know it doesn't hurt. Children who are thus empowered are more confident about new experiences. Children who are more cautious will want to stop often, simply to reassure themselves that they still have control. As you will see, giving children this veto power has been critical to the success of our dental practice.

Modeling from Other Children

Young children learn by watching others. For most, it is then easy and natural to do the same thing. Mimicking is an instinctive ability that all children have, and most are very good at it from infancy on. In the beginning, they copy their parents and later, their older siblings and other children. My guess is that this is another one of those instincts that favors survival.

We can take advantage of this instinct in the dental office by allowing uninitiated children to observe more experienced ones. Seeing is believing. First, a child observes another who is in no obvious distress and then it is their turn.

The unknown can be frightening for a child. The known is predictable. If another child is not available, a favorite doll or stuffed animal will work. Before we do anything with the child, we do a dry run on the doll first, then tell the child, "Okay, now it's your turn." Psychologists call this "modeling." Apprehensive and cautious children may need to observe on a number of occasions or observe several different children to be convinced that there is no danger.

A Customized Pace

The parents and the dentist both need to be flexible and willing to pace the treatment according to the child's response rather than the adults' agenda. Just as children respond individually to local anesthesia, they will respond differently to the whole dental experience. Some children are able to have four restorations done at one sitting while others need four sittings for one restoration.

Individual differences need to be noticed and respected, even in small children. In our office, notes in the child's chart help us remember such things as "Needed double anesthetic" or "Do everything on her doll first" or "Behavior better with Aunt Sue or Grandpa Joe" or "Short appointments only."

Progressive Desensitization

When a child is afraid of something, that fear can be comfortably conquered if it is gradually confronted. Simply being in a dental office can be frightening for some children, especially if they have already had a bad dental experience. If that is the case, then the child can be brought to the office for a few minutes, have a look around, and then leave. As they look around, if they see pleasant things, coming back and doing it again will be less frightening. During the second trip, on another day or even later the same day, the child can play some games, watch a video, pick out a toy, and then leave. In fact, we carry this idea of progressive desensitization into our whole practice (see Appendix II for a detailed scenario of how we do this).

While this process may seem unnecessarily time-consuming, when we consider the long-term consequences of dental trauma, dental phobia, and neglected teeth, it becomes worth the effort. For most children, this process of progressive desensitization occurs quite rapidly, but for all children, offering the process can lead to a calm and happy time in your office.

The First Visit for an Apprehensive Child

The first thing we need to do is get the child into the chair without scaring them. If there is another child having something done nearby, we point to them and say, "Look. Now it is your turn." As we say this, we gently lift the child into the chair. It's not good to ask the child if she wants to get up in the chair because if she says no, there is not much you can do without pleading or force, and these are not good alternatives. If there is no other child to look at, a doll can be used as an example. Then we simply say, as we lift her up, "Come and sit on this chair." It's never a question; rather, it's a statement in a tone of voice that implies this is not a big deal, that it is a normal, ordinary thing.

If the child seems a little afraid or still uneasy, we position her so that she is sitting up sideways with her legs hanging over the side, instead of having her lie down right away. Then after a few moments, we help her to lean back. If there is resistance, we don't fight it. We simply wait a few seconds and try again. Occasionally, their first prophy is done sitting up. If restorations are needed, we send anxious children home with a scented nitrous oxide nasal hood so they can practice.

The Anxiety Reduction Program (ARP)

The cleaning appointment is relatively non-threatening and fairly well tolerated by most children. However, if that simple procedure evokes a fearful response, it is likely that having a restoration will be even more problematic. Instead of pushing on through, we gradually work up to it over a few short visits. Each visit is fast and not expensive. We call this the "anxiety reduction program" or ARP.

Here's how it works. On a separate appointment, the child is shown a standard set-up for a restoration. This can include the nitrous oxide set-up, a cotton applicator, a syringe without needle, a high-speed dental hand piece without bur, a low-speed hand piece with a medium-sized round bur, a dental mirror, and a burnisher.

Next, the assistant gently touches each instrument on her own fingertips, then without saying a word, she touches them to the child's fingers. If the child is afraid and withdraws her hand, the assistant will allow her that freedom but then will gently and immediately try again.

Once the child has verified that she has the freedom to withdraw her hand at will, she will be less afraid because she has been given some control. We often tell children in our practice: "You're the boss. While you are here in my office, I'll let you be the boss, but at home your mother and father are the boss." They almost always smile when we say that and usually test us a few times just to be sure. They love the power.

When the hand pieces are introduced through finger touching the first time, they are not running. The second time, they are running so the child can hear the noise and feel the vibration in his fingers. We always touch each of our own fingers and each of the child's fingers with each instrument we intend to use. That way, there are no surprises; nothing happens to violate trust. In fact, a bond of trust is being non-verbally developed.

Next, we do the same thing again, only this time we touch the front teeth with each instrument including the hand pieces. Then the nosepiece for nitrous oxide is introduced without hoses at first. Then hoses are added and a mixture of 50 percent nitrous oxide and 50 percent oxygen is given for 90 seconds as a rehearsal for the next visit.

The key to ARP is to not advance to the next level until the previous one is comfortably accomplished. The sequence for an ARP visit in our office is often as follows:

1. Sit in the chair.

2. Lie down.

3. Air, water, vacuum-paper cup, palm of hand, mouth.

4. Rubber cup-fingers-teeth.

5. Doctor exam-mirror + air.

6. Nasal N_2O hood w/out hoses.

7. Nasal N_2O hood w/hoses.

8. N_2O/O_2, 50/50, 90 seconds.

9. Pretend topical cotton applicator.

10. Pretend injection syringe without needle.

11. Low-speed hand piece fingers/teeth.

12. High-speed hand piece fingers/teeth.

13. Rubber dam on finger.

14. Matrix on finger.

Several ARP visits may be needed. Our fee is $35 per visit, which makes it affordable. Insurance does not typically cover these visits. My personal time is about 2 minutes and the remaining 18 minutes are with an assistant. When parents understand the difference of costs between the hospital and ARP, they usually prefer the latter. Roughly only half of one percent of our restorative patients go to the hospital.

Alternative Restorative Treatment (ART) and Medical Caries Arrestment (MCA) are also sometimes used to delay definitive treatments (see below). Force is never an option. We have no quiet room or restraining devices, and crying almost never occurs.

The Child Is the Boss

If at any time the child seems hesitant, we simply say, "Remember, you are the boss. If you want me to give you a rest, just raise your hand like this." As we say this, we gently help her raise her hand so she can see what we mean. To verify that she understands and really is in control, we then say, "Now show me what you are going to do if you want me to stop and give you a rest." This time she must raise her hand on her own. If she doesn't, we show her again—and again—until she has it. This gives the child the all-important power of choice.

In our experience, the children love this power, and most do not abuse it. Of course, some very cautious children will raise their hand frequently at first just to verify that we are going do what we said. We know that if we fail that test, trust is lost and fear returns. So we honor this promise at all times: "Okay, Boss, can I do a little more?" However, if we suspect the signal is not being taken seriously, we'll say, "If you keep doing that, we'll never get done" or "I'm going to have to get your mother!"

Fearful children need frequent, short breaks, often just a minute or two. It's not uncommon for us to say, "You did such a good job of getting up on the chair. Jump down and get another toy. Then we'll do it again in a minute."

Control of Pain

Pain should neither be ignored nor its importance diminished. Pain—and the dentist's failure to respond appropriately to it—is the single most important reason why roughly 20% of the people in this country fear the dentist. When a woman giving birth experiences pain, nature helps her forget it, but when a child experiences pain at the dentist, it may be remembered for many years. If the dentist and staff take the necessary time and use the best available techniques and medications, there is no reason why any child should have to endure pain. Nitrous oxide and a painless injection technique (see Appendix III) are essential.

In addition, some children have an atypical body chemistry or nerve anatomy. These individuals can have a hard time getting numb. They may need extra anesthetic or a special type of injection. When a child says, "It still hurts," we always believe them and stop immediately even when we've given more than enough anesthetic.

Pain must be avoided, even if it means stopping the procedure in the middle and trying on another day. The important issue is that we want the child to grow up feeling good about dentistry. To have this happen, both dentist and parent must be uncompromisingly committed to a pleasant experience for the child. Neither pain nor force can be an option.

A Word about Drugs

For me, nitrous oxide works very well. It's safe and effective. Sedatives and tranquilizers, however, were never as predictable in my hands. They seemed to work about 50% of the time. Whether they worked or not, I usually pushed on through and finished the case. It was not fun. On the next visit, I would usually increase the dose. Some of those kids were hard to wake up. Even with the reversal drugs loaded and ready to go, it made me nervous. Eventually, because of inconsistent results and fear of overdose, I stopped using them all together.

General Anesthesia

A gentle attempt should be made to repair one tooth using normal dental office methods before the decision is made to use general anesthesia. If the decay is not severe, that attempt should also include non-drilling methods of temporarily treating decay by the methods described in the next chapter. If the damage to the teeth is too far advanced or if the parent is not willing or able to make the necessary changes regarding fluoride, sweets, and frequency of dental visits, then general anesthesia is the best choice.

7

PARENTS, PERSONALITIES, AND PROCEDURES

Besides eliminating pain and giving the child control in the dental chair, other considerations can help create a dental experience that is free from fear.

Put the Parent at Ease

As we've seen, many parents transmit their own dental fears to their children without realizing it. They may not actually say to the child, "Look out! The dentist will hurt you." But their tone of voice, facial expressions, and gestures all warn the child of danger.

Children are very experienced at reading their parent's nonverbal cues; after all, they have been doing it since infancy—long before they used language. So if one or both parents have had a bad childhood experience at the dentist, they will naturally be concerned and even uneasy that the same thing may happen again, this time to their child. Such concern is easily noticed by the child.

The dentist must reassure the parent that, above all else, their child will always leave the office with a good memory of their dental experience, even if it means stopping in the middle of a procedure and trying again on another day.

Personality Types

Lots of things influence a child's personality: genetics, life experiences, and even birth order. Some children are bold and jump headfirst into everything new, while others are shy and cautious. If a shy child is pushed too hard, the shyness will become even more pronounced and the needed rapport with the dentist and his team will be even more difficult to establish.

Birth Order

When two siblings go to a new dentist for the first time, frequently the younger one is more willing to meet the dentist and explore the office. One would think that the older, more experienced child would be more willing but, in fact, the opposite is often true.

Why is this the case? The first child in a family always gets noticed because they are the only show in town. Doting parents lavish lots of attention on the first-born as they learn to be parents. The second (and any subsequent) child must share attention, must learn to be creative so as to stand out and divert parental attention from the first child. This makes the younger siblings by necessity more accustomed to trying new things and even more comfortable with them. When possible, we find it works well to schedule both children for the same day and let the younger one go first if the older is hesitant.

Delaying Conventional Treatment with Medical Caries Arrestment (MCA) or Alternative Restorative Treatment (ART)

As you know, all decay is not the same. Some forms are more aggressive than others. When decay is very soft, it is light brown in color and spreads relatively quickly; this is "active" decay. But when it is harder and almost black, it barely progresses at all. This condition we know as "arrested" decay.

If your goal is to safely delay dental repairs until a child is old enough to tolerate anxiety-free treatment, the process requires converting the decay from active to arrested. This can be done medically instead of surgically. It is good for the child and good for the dentist and saves the parent the expense associated with hospital dental treatment.

Medical caries arrestment (MCA), as I call it, is the non-surgical treatment of dental caries; it typically consists of a combination of dietary changes combined with the topical application of various substances such as fluoride varnish, chlorohexidine, or iodine every 2–3 months[1].

MCA is not for everyone. Some younger children with advanced decay in multiple teeth that are already abscessed, or soon to abscess, may not be good candidates. These children need immediate definitive treatment, using either effective sedation or general anesthesia. Early or moderately advanced decay, however, can be slowed down or stopped using medical or non-surgical methods for a long enough period to allow the child to mature sufficiently to comfortably tolerate conventional treatment in the dental office.

If, for any reason, the non-surgical methods are not effective and the decay fails to arrest, immediate definitive treatment may be needed. It should be remembered that in no case should a terrified, screaming child be restrained for treatment due to the potential long-term ill effects. It is simply not worth the risk because we cannot know in advance which children will become dental phobics.

Numerous solutions are used for MCA. In fact, this is the subject of much discussion. Fluoride varnish, 1% chlorohexidine, 10% povidone iodine, and silver diamine fluoride are all currently in clinical trials. While the official jury is still out, I have used fluoride varnish every three months for the last eight years with good success. Recently, we added iodine. In combination with parental involvement at home with

---

1. Milgrom P, Weinstein P. *Early Childhood Caries.* University of Washington Press: Seattle, WA, 1999; 66-67.

diet and application of fluoride toothpaste four times each day, it is remarkable how many lesions have been arrested and how many "untreatable" children have been treated successfully. (See Appendices IV & V for examples of parent handouts.)

Alternative restorative treatment (ART) also has a place. The details of this technique are available from the World Health Organization and a number of journal articles[2], but a simple description will suffice here. ART involves the scraping away of superficial decay using hand instruments instead of a hand piece. The peripheral decay at the Cavo-surface Junction must be scraped down to sound dentin, but the central portion over the pulp can be left in place. I use a small spoon excavator. A glass ionomer filling is then placed. A good peripheral seal is best. Later when the child is a little older and able to tolerate conventional treatment, the filling can be redone using conventional methods.

Even an abscessed tooth can be temporarily treated by less invasive means. A tiny hole can be painlessly drilled in the offending tooth, thus draining the pressure. Combining draining with antibiotics gives the dentist and the child time. Over a few short weeks and some ARP visits, the child can be gently prepared for the treatment needed.

Dentists have used a variant of ART for years when they placed small orthodontic bands on primary anterior incisors. It still works, especially when cemented with glass ionomer. Scrape away superficial decay with a spoon, and cement a band, knee to knee. No injection, no hand piece, no struggle. A year or two later, a more esthetic restoration can be placed in the office.

What about lost income?

If you practice my methods as described here, your income from the restorative dentistry portion of your practice might go down at first. But there are many benefits—both short-term and long-term—to what I've learned to do.

2.   Frencken JE, Holmgren CJ. ART: A minimal intervention approach to managing dental caries. *Dent Update* 2004 June;31(5):295-298, 301.

First, both parental satisfaction and your blood pressure are going to benefit right away. I used to worry about production, about using my time the most efficiently. The old voice control and restraint techniques fit right in. But when I made a commitment to having a no-fear practice, I started scheduling children with behavior issues differently, i.e., in very short appointments until each child demonstrated that he could sit quietly during a bigger block of my time. That way, if patients went home with nothing done, it wasn't much out of my time or income. I began charging a nominal fee for anxiety-reduction visits, always talking to the parents from the beginning about the need to go slow with a particular child who was afraid. Few of the parents ever objected; most were very relieved to have someone who cared about the feelings of their child first.

Over the years, my income, inflation-adjusted, has gone up as parent satisfaction has gone up. When the word got out in the community that our patients were happy and not afraid, it was more profitable than all the expensive advertising available.

Quality of life is another issue. As you can imagine, office stress levels have gone way down. I enjoy coming to work rather than trying to let difficult patients "run off my back." Now there is nothing to run off except the occasional person who doesn't pay their bill. What's more, I'm not anxious to retire because coming to work is easy and fun.

Trying a different way

If your education included physical restraints and or crying rooms like mine did, I invite you to experiment with a new approach.

1. First, decide that you would like to try methods that involve no harsh words or force. Tell yourself that you are concerned that the child might grow up with a long-lasting bad memory of the dentist and that you want to try a gentler approach.

2. If at the time of the first visit, you realize that the child may have behavior issues, tell the parents that their child will need extra

time: time to watch other children, time to practice and pretend. Then they will know what to expect and why and they will know it ahead of time, not after. Make sure it is a short appointment so if you get nothing done, neither you nor the parent will have wasted much time.

3. Try treating dental caries medically with MCA or with ART rather than conventional surgical methods on those children who are behaviorally challenged.

4. Try the painless 2-step injection method described in Appendix III.

5. We often get so focused on a task that we miss subtle patient cues, so ask your assistant to silently signal you by a touch on your shoulder if she thinks the child needs a rest.

6. If things are going downhill, stop right away. Don't wait until the child cries. Then try again soon, but try something easy. Build confidence.

7. Remember, you are not the parent. You cannot be responsible for parental neglect or inability. Don't make their problems your problems. Refuse to use force. If they don't accept that, it's their problem, not yours.

What if things don't go as planned?

What if a child refuses to do anything, in spite of all your efforts to be kind and gentle, in spite of observing other children and rehearsal visits? What then? Is there ever a time when simply holding the child down and getting treatment completed is justified?

The answer is no. The potential long-term consequences of a violent act, for that's what it is, outweigh the benefits. Force should never be an option.

Certainly, if nothing at all is working and non-surgical treatment of decay or ART is inappropriate, a general anesthetic is the best option. If for any reason, hospital treatment is not possible, consider a referral to an oral surgeon who can simply remove the diseased teeth under general anesthesia.

8

TIMES HAVE CHANGED

It is time for a fresh look at how we do things. It is time for us to recognize that we are not obligated to treat children who will not allow it. It is time for us to realize that even when pushed by parents, clinic managers, or our own egos, we do more harm than good when we treat children against their will. It is time for us to stop using force in spite of what has been acceptable in the past. It is time for us to spend less time covering our behinds with all-inclusive informed consent documents and more time figuring out ways to do things in such a way that children remember dentists as being kind, gentle, and safe people. Aversive conditioning needs to become an embarrassing footnote in dental history.

The phobic patient's cycle of avoidance, abscess, and extraction can be broken by treating children in such a way that they have good dental memories and want to come back. The 30 million phobic adults in this country are living proof that we need to change the way we get things done.

APPENDIX A

WHAT TO SAY TO YOUR CHILD

Parents frequently ask us, "What should I say to my child before going to the dentist?"

WHAT TO SAY:

Tomorrow we're going to the dentist. The dentist helps us make sure your teeth stay strong and healthy. You'll get a new toothbrush and two toys. Then your teeth will get polished and coated with marshmallow or bubble gum fluoride.

WHAT NOT TO SAY:

Tomorrow you have to go to the dentist. I want you to be good and not move around while you are having your teeth checked. Don't worry about anything because it won't hurt.

HOW TO ANSWER QUESTIONS:

It's natural for a child to ask questions, but the answers, and the way they are phrased, can get tricky. It's simplest if you write your child's questions down and ask us when you get here.

WHAT WILL HAPPEN WHILE YOU ARE HERE:

When you arrive at the office, I will come out to the reception room to greet you. A simple, nonverbal, get-acquainted routine has been designed to give your child a sense of well-being. We'll develop a relationship based on friendliness and trust rather than on authority. If your child feels a sense of self-control, there will be no fear.

During this portion of the visit, if you try to help, it may have the opposite effect, so please remain a silent partner. Your physical presence alone is all that is needed to reassure your child that all is well. Children are very good at reading their parents' feelings and non-verbal cues. If you are relaxed, your child will be too. If you read a magazine while we are getting acquainted with your child, you will be showing that there's no cause for alarm.

Next, you'll both get a guided tour of the office. One of our highlights will be meeting and feeding the animals. (We have live gerbils in a cage.) Again, try to remain in the background and continue being a silent partner. When your child is ready, we'll move on to the cleaning, fluoride application, and examination.

Usually things go smoothly, but occasionally a child becomes apprehensive. If this happens, we don't push. The goal is to have your child feel comfortable coming to the dentist. We'll do whatever is necessary to achieve that goal, even if it means spoiling them a little. Eventually, they come around.

Looking forward to meeting you both.

Appendix B

THE APPREHENSIVE CHILD: A CASE STUDY

The following scenario is a typical series of visits in our office of an apprehensive child.

The Meeting

The silent intercom light on the wall blinks and I know that our next new patient has arrived. "Try not to keep them waiting," I think. "It makes a bad first impression."

I walk out to the reception room where there are several parents that I know. We exchange smiles and greetings as I walk by. I move quickly to the far end of the room to the receptionist, who hands me the new patient's medical and dental history and a blank chart in a folder. Glancing over the history quickly, I see that we have a 3-year-old boy named Steven who has already been to the dentist once. Under the section on previous dental care is written this: "Would not let the dentist work on him."

Not wanting to alarm the child, I call out the mother's name. "Mrs. Rose?"

As I glance around the room, a sober-faced woman in her mid-30s stands up, grasps her son's wrist firmly, and says, "I'm Mrs. Rose."

I walk over to her and introduce myself, and we shake hands. Without speaking directly to the child, I extend my hand to him as I had just done to his mother. Shunning this non-verbal gesture, he darts behind his mother. I don't comment or pursue him. Other than that one brief effort to befriend the child, this initial encounter in the reception room focuses on the parent. If too much attention is paid to the child during these early moments, he may become suspicious. However, in an effort to empower the boy and thus allay any anxiety he may have, I ask, "Steven, can I talk to your mother for a minute?"

He blinks his eyes and nods.

"I notice your boy is a little shy," I say to Mrs. Rose.

"Oh yes, he's always been that way in new situations," says the mother. "Sometimes he's even that way with his own grandparents."

"Some kids are just born that way. They're naturally shy," I say.

"I know," she says, "I think that's what went wrong at the last dentist. They didn't take enough time with him, and it was all downhill from there. They just jumped right in and tried to do a cleaning and it scared him."

I nod. "Mrs. Rose, I know from experience that these first impressions really do last a long time, so for that reason I promise you that I'll bend over backwards to make sure your son has a good time here today. It's very important that he grow up feeling good about going to the dentist. I'll do whatever it takes, even if I have to spoil him. Is that okay with you?"

She smiles warmly, "I'm so very glad to hear that. I've really been dreading this."

At the same time, I notice her releasing the death grip on her son's wrist. He instinctively senses her relaxation and begins playing with a toy truck a few feet away.

"Have you noticed anything in his mouth that you're wondering about?" I inquire softly.

"Yes," she whispers, "I think he's got a cavity on his lower back molar."

"Any pain?" I ask.

"No, but I was hoping you could fix it today because I had to take time off from work."

"I'll sure do my best," I answer, "but we need to be careful not to do anything that would scare him for years to come. Is that okay with you?"

"Oh yes, I don't want him to be afraid like I am when he grows up. I had an awful time when I was in the second grade. I still remember it. He was such a mean dentist. He actually yelled at me and told my mother to go out to the waiting room. She got so mad at him that she just picked me up and took me home."

"I'm sorry you had such a bad experience," I reply, "and I'm glad your mother stuck up for you. Come and let me show you around our office."

The Tour

As we start walking from the reception room toward the clinic, it becomes obvious that her son does not want to go. She prods Steven to follow us.

"Oh, that's okay," I say. "The tour is mainly for you. He can stay out here if he wants."

Her son crosses his arms and sits down belligerently. I coach Mrs. Rose to not look back; then she and I slowly walk away and begin the tour.

"On your right is the hygiene area. That's where every six months the children get their cleanings, fluoride treatments, sealants, and dietary advice. We place a lot of emphasis on prevention because in the long run, it's so much better for the children. And it's easier on the parents and us too."

As I'm talking to Mrs. Rose, I notice Steven peering curiously from the reception room. I make no effort to encourage him to come in, because if I did, he'd probably run the other way. I advise his mother to do the same. She complies with some difficulty.

"Around this corner," I say as I continue walking with his mother, "is the video room where children can watch cartoons and movies while they wait for their brothers and sisters. And over here are the video games. We have both Nintendo and three Game Boys."

Steven has now cautiously walked in and stands silently next to his mother, holding on to her dress with one hand and sucking his thumb with the other. I softly instruct his mother, "Try to ignore him."

As we continue straight ahead, I point to a small cage on the floor a few feet away. "Mrs. Rose, those are our gerbils."

In the cage two gerbils are romping around on a bed of wood shavings. "Does your boy like animals?"

"Oh yes, we've got two dogs at home and he loves them."

Overhearing us, Steven now notices the gerbils and our hygienist Jamie, who is intentionally seated on the floor next to the cage. She is feeding the gerbils by dropping sunflower seeds through the mesh screen cover. Jamie gestures for Steven to join her. He does so without hesitation and she gives him some seeds. This entire transaction is nonverbal, an important technique when getting to know a preschooler. Jamie hands him a few more seeds. He takes them and continues feeding. They are developing rapport.

I continue the tour with Mrs. Rose. "Over here is my private office," I point to my small stand-up desk. "I used to have a whole room, but we needed the space. So all I get now is this," I say with a smile. Mrs. Rose laughs and turns around to see how her son is doing. He's totally focused on the gerbils and obviously in no distress. Jamie makes sure he's got a steady supply of seeds. "Over here is the door to the staff lounge, next to that is the x-ray darkroom, and around the corner over here is the x-ray room."

As we walk around the corner and out of her son's view, I explain, "This wasn't always the x-ray room. In fact, it used to be the crying room. The entranceway that you're standing in right now used to have a soundproof door. My methods of treating children were different in those days. The whole philosophy was different. It was more of an authoritarian approach, but I don't use that approach anymore. Now we empower children and allow them to feel like they have some control over what happens to them. We let them watch other children having treatment so they can see with their own eyes that no harm will come. Then we begin slowly with easy things first and build their confidence step by step. It is called 'progressive desensitization.' And finally, we make sure nothing hurts." Then Mrs. Rose and I talk about nitrous oxide and painless injections.

I notice Mrs. Rose looking over her shoulder for Steven. I realize that she is probably worrying about him because he has been out of her sight for a few minutes. "I wonder how your son is doing," I say to her.

"I do too," she says. I follow her out of the room. Steven and Jamie are both gone from the gerbil area. She turns and asks me, "Where are they?"

"They're around," I reply. "Let's find out."

We look around and see him way down at the far end of the long hygiene room. Steven is lying down in the treatment chair, in no obvious distress. Jamie is now cleaning his teeth.

"I can't believe my eyes! He's obviously okay with it," she says with surprise.

"Jamie's very good at what she does," I tell her. "As long as everything is going so well, why don't we just leave them alone? If we go over there, it may change the dynamics. Are you okay with that?"

"Yes, certainly, I don't want to spoil what's going on. I'm so relieved," she says as she dabs her eyes with a tissue.

Advice to the Parent

"Let's go out to the reception room where I will have my assistant Michelle go over some things with you that will help Steven avoid cavities," I say to Mrs. Rose. We then head on out to the front of the office.

"By the way, Mrs. Rose," I say. "As we walk back out through the clinical section, don't say anything to Steven or even look at him as we go by. If you do, he may misinterpret your interest and think you are concerned about him. Then he might panic and want to leave. You can glance out of the corner of your eye, but don't let him catch you look-ing or this whole thing could fall apart."

The mother plays her part perfectly and we walk back out to the reception room. I ask Mrs. Rose to sit down with Michelle and say, "While I go in and check on Steven, Michelle will go over some impor-tant material on cavity prevention with you. Do you have any ques-tions before I go?"

"Yes, Doctor, how long before he will be done? Can I go back to see him?"

"Oh, I'd say about 15 minutes. Of course, you're free to go back anytime you wish, but if he notices you looking at him, his good behavior might change. So if you do go back there, just peek around the corner to satisfy your curiosity and then go back to the reception room, okay?"

She smiles and nods in agreement.

"Okay," I say, "when Jamie is done with the cleaning, she'll come out and get you because we want you to be there when we do the examination."

As I leave the room to check on Steven, Michelle begins explaining some important things to his mother about cavity prevention and den-tal health

The Cleaning

While Mrs. Rose and I had been on the tour, Steven and Jamie had been sitting by the toys and gerbils.

"Steven," says Jamie, "now that you've fed the gerbils and picked out your first toy, I want to see your teeth. Can you open your mouth really wide? That's it! Wow, you've got nice teeth! But it's not very light in here. Let's go over to the other room where there is more light."

Assuming willingness and compliance, Jamie extends her fingers for Steven to take as an assist in getting up off the floor. As they walk from the toy box to the treatment area, they pass another child lying on a treatment chair having a cleaning.

"Look, Steven," says Jamie, "see how wide he can open his mouth?"

Once they reach Jamie's station, she says, "Here's your place! Jump up so I can see your teeth better. That's it—wow, you've got beautiful teeth, but there's a piece of food on this one. I'll get it off with this toothbrush. There, that's nice. But wait! There's still a little piece left—let me use my electric toothbrush. Listen to how it sounds when I touch it on my finger. Now let's try it on your finger. Sort of tickles, doesn't it?"

After showing Steven the motor-driven rubber cup and touching it to his finger so he can get an idea of what it will feel like, Jamie proceeds. "Now I'll tickle your tooth to get it clean, and we'll use this special bubble-gum-flavored toothpaste. That's beautiful—let's do them all!"

Before she proceeds, she says, "Steven, while I'm tickling your teeth, if you want to rest, just raise your hand like this." She gently lifts up his arm to demonstrate. "Now show me what you're going to do if you want to rest."

When Steven lifts his hand, she says, "That's it! Perfect! I'll let you be the boss." And she proceeds quietly and easily into a full cleaning. Well trained in the gentle approach, Jamie knows that if Steven does raise his hand, she will stop and then adjust the pace, for example, spending more time cleaning the anteriors before proceeding to the molars.

As she finishes, she says, "Wow, Steven, they look wonderful! Your mother's going to be so proud. There, now all your teeth are clean. Now, let's clean in between your teeth with dental floss."

When that's done, she says, "Next I'm going to brush them with special marshmallow fluoride gel for three minutes to make them strong. Then it'll be time to go pick out another toy." She brushes on the flavored fluoride and simultaneously vacuums off the excess.

"Mmmm, doesn't that taste good? While I'm brushing it on, I'll tell you a little story of *Goldilocks and the Three Bears*."

After the fluoride treatment, Jamie notifies her assistant that she is ready for Mrs. Rose and the doctor. She tells Steven, "They're going to look at your beautiful teeth and then you get another toy and then go home. Here they come! Aren't you excited?"

The Examination

"Excuse me, Mrs. Rose," Jamie's assistant interrupts the conversation between Michelle and Steven's mother. "It's time to come in the other room so you can be there while Steven's teeth are being examined. When we go in there, try to be our silent partner so that Doctor can tell you everything he notices in Steven's mouth. There will be lots of time for talking when he is done." She then escorts Mrs. Rose to the seat next to her son's dental chair.

"Hi again, Mrs. Rose," I say. "Steven's been doing a wonderful job, and as soon as I am done looking at his teeth, he will be able to get up and talk. Let me just read off what I see in his mouth to Jamie. Look how wide he is opening his mouth! Let's see. His gums look wonderful, his bite is excellent, but I do see a cavity. Fortunately, you brought him in soon enough so repairing it should be uncomplicated. But because he is so young and because he had a scary time the last time he went to the dentist, we will need to be extra careful to make sure he remembers it as a good experience. We both want him to grow up feeling good about going to the dentist, right?"

"Yes, of course, Doctor Pike." Steven's mother agrees. "How should we go about that?"

"We do that by making sure we get our priorities right. The first priority is always the child and his memory of the dentist. The second is the repair of the tooth. We know that two things will create a bad memory: fear and pain. To be sure that he has a good experience, we first go through a rehearsal sequence designed to eliminate the fear.

Then and only then will we repair his tooth in such a way that he feels no pain.

"Eliminating the fear involves two steps. First, he will watch other children while they get dental work done and then he will personally experience a pretend filling, a dress rehearsal, so to speak. We will show him all the instruments one by one, the drill, the syringe, even the laughing gas. This is that progressive desensitization I told you about. We will even have him breathe a little laughing gas just so he will know how it feels.

"If one of the instruments has moving parts that make a sound or vibration, we will show him first on our fingers, then on his fingers, and finally on his tooth. If he seems anxious, we will let him know that he is the boss and we won't do anything if he says no. We will tell him to raise his hand if he wants to stop.

"Most children love that power and usually test it a few times just to be sure we will do what we say. Once they have tested us and verified it a few times, things usually go well unless we do something that violates the agreement. We are very careful to keep our promise no matter what. Our credibility, the child's trust, and our rapport are more important than anything. If we are in a hurry to get done and violate the trust by pushing on through, then the child may get his tooth fixed, but he will also have learned that dentists can't be trusted. The battle will be won but the war will be lost."

I continue. "After Steven has watched other children getting their dental work done, and after he has had a dress rehearsal, he will be ready for the filling. As long as it doesn't hurt and he feels like he is in control, everything emotionally should be fine."

"Well, I understand the part of his raising his hand if he wants to rest and be in control and all that, but what about the pain?" Mrs. Rose asks. "Some things just hurt, like the shot, for instance."

"I'm glad you asked. We've found that if we pay attention to detail and take the time, then things can be done with no pain and no use of force. If for any reason what we do here is not working, we always have the option of a general anesthetic or some of the alternative non-surgical techniques. When you come back next week, you can watch from a distance while we do the rehearsal so you can see with your own eyes how smoothly this goes. Come, I'll walk you out to the desk so we can set up his rehearsal appointment."

As he walks out, 3-year-old Steven seems very happy. He has got a new toothbrush and two toys, and everybody's been nice to him. It is hard to believe that only 45 minutes ago he was sitting in the reception room with his arms folded and refusing to follow his mother.

The Rehearsal Visit

The following week Steven and Mrs. Rose return, but this time things are different. As his mother opens the door, Steven pushes on by her and runs through the reception room and back to the toy box.

Michelle and Jamie greet him. "Hi, Steven, we are going to have fun today. First it's time to pick out a toy and then just before you leave, we'll get another one."

While he is picking out a toy, his mother walks in and Michelle quietly comments to Mrs. Rose, "As long as things are going so well, why don't you go out and sit down in the reception room? If he wants you, we will come and get you right away. You may not get another chance to sit down and read a magazine until he is asleep tonight," she says with a laugh. "If you say anything to him as you walk out, he will likely get nervous so just ignore him completely."

As soon as Steven has picked out a toy, Michelle gently takes him by the hand and walks him over to another child who is undergoing treatment. "Steven, look how still Marney is holding her arms and legs. And look how good she is and how big she is opening her mouth. Okay, now it is your turn. Jump up here and you will see how easy it is." As she is saying this, she gently lifts him up.

Now he is sitting sidesaddle on the dental chair. "Steven, let's put your feet up here," she says as she lifts his feet and places them on the footrest. "There! That's wonderful. Now lay your head down on the soft pillow, just like Marney over there. That's right. I've got some great things to show you and then you get to pick out another toy.

"First, look at all these nice things that help me look at your teeth." She touches the dental mirror on her own gloved fingers, then on his fingers, and then on his front teeth. Testing his authority, he pushes her hand away. Instantly she stops touching his teeth and goes back to demonstrating on his fingers. Then in a second or two she tries again. This time he permits it. She does not move on to the second instrument until he is okay with the first one. In this way, Michelle goes through all the instruments and various items including the hand pieces.

The last item is the soft, scented nasal hood used for the nitrous oxide. It has no hoses attached. Instead of touching it on his teeth, she touches it on his chin, then his ear, and finally his nose. She leaves it gently resting on his nose for about 10 seconds so he can get used to it.

"Steven," she says, "you are wonderful. Now we have got one last thing to do before you get up and get another toy, and you are going to love it because it makes you laugh." At this point, Michelle motions for Jamie to come over. As a hygienist, Jamie is trained and licensed to administer nitrous oxide. Steven's already familiar with Jamie because she cleaned his teeth on the earlier visit.

Jamie attaches the hoses to the scented nasal hood and gently places it on his nose without saying a word. He doesn't protest because he just did it a few seconds ago. First she turns on the oxygen alone and then adds the nitrous oxide until the ratio is 50/50. As a distraction, she tells a story. The whole thing takes under two minutes. Like most 3-year-olds, Steven loves a story. After the short exposure to nitrous oxide and oxygen, he is wide awake and smiling broadly.

"How did you like that?" Jamie says as she turns off the gas and removes the hood.

"Fine," Steven says, in a very relaxed, slow drawl.

"That's wonderful," Jamie says "Let me finish a little more of the story and then it will be time to get up and get another toy. You are wonderful."

After another minute or two of storytelling, the effects of the nitrous oxide are gone and Jamie says, "Michelle, Steven's ready to pick out another toy now. Will you please go with him?"

Steven runs ahead of Michelle to the toy box. "Let's go out and show your mother what you picked out," Michelle says.

Steven runs out to show his mother, who has been peeking in from the other room. She is delighted. "Did everything go okay?" she inquires.

"Oh, yes, he did a wonderful job," says Michelle. "When you come back next time, he will know what to expect."

"Do I need to prepare him for the shot and the drilling?" Mrs. Rose asks.

"No," says Michelle, "it will be best if you don't say anything. If he does ask any questions, just write them down and we will go over them next visit. If you try to answer his questions, your answer could be different from ours and that might confuse him. Remember that we want to all be on the same page here. We want him to grow up with a good memory of the dentist. Come, let's get an appointment for his filling."

The Filling

When Steven returns for his filling, he again comes bounding in. Again he is welcomed by Michelle and Jamie. He picks out a toy and jumps up in the chair enthusiastically.

Jamie explains to him what is going to happen. "Steven, remember last time when you had that soft thing on your nose and it made you feel like laughing? Well, we're going to do it again. Want to hear another story?"

When Steven nods, she says. "Here we go."

Without hesitation Jamie gently places the nasal hood on his nose, holds it snug to his skin so there are no leaks, adjusts the flow of oxygen and nitrous oxide, and begins telling a story. "Once upon a time there were three bears…"

Again, as she begins the story, she slips the hood to the side for a second, dries the tissue with cotton, and applies a speck of cherry-flavored topical anesthetic, then replaces the hood. The story continues without pause. After about 90 seconds, she removes the hood and turns off the flow of gas. Steven is smiling.

Continuing with the story, Jamie places a few drops of citanist plain just below the surface of his tissue with a .30 gauge extra-short needle; his expression hardly changes. The story continues. After two or three minutes and using more nitrous oxide, she injects the xylocaine or septocaine.

"Steven," she says, "pretty soon your mouth is going to feel funny, so don't be surprised. It will feel like fairies are dancing on your lip. Can you feel them? Later today, they'll go away. Let's go pick out another toy and play for a few minutes."

Michelle comes over and plays too. When about ten minutes have passed, Michelle says, "Steven, come back to the chair, please. I want to look at your teeth."

They go back to the chair, she helps him climb up, and she looks at his teeth. With surprise, she says, "Oh my goodness, I think I see a germ in your tooth. Doctor, come take a look at this."

On cue, I join them and look in Steven's mouth. "Yes, Michelle, I see it. It looks like it's trying to eat Steven's tooth."

"Oh my, Doctor, can you help us get that bad bug out of Steven's tooth?"

"I'd be glad to," I say. "My two helpers, Mr. Whistle [high-speed drill] and Mr. Bumpy [slow-speed drill] can get him out."

Steven and I rehearse the hand-raising technique that lets him know that he's the boss.

"That's it, Steven, hold your mouth open wide so I can get him out of your tooth. Good job! I've got him!"

"Oh, wonderful," says Michelle. "Now I can see a hole in Steven's tooth where the bug used to live. We don't want another bug to crawl in there! What should we do, Doctor?"

"Let's fill it up with sour cream," I say. "Look. I've got some right here," and I squirt a small drop of white filling material (Fugi IX, Fugi II, or Photac) on Michelle's finger and then on Steven's.

"What a great idea, Doctor!" says Michelle. "Hurry up before another bug goes in there."

"Ok, I'll do it right away," I say. "Let me shine my flashlight on it so I can see what I'm doing." Then I cure the material and smooth it down. "Okay, Steven, time to get up and pick out another toy!"

Michelle then says, "Steven, we have to wait for the dancing fairies to leave so if you bite on this soft pillow [a dental cotton roll] they'll have room to go home. Your mother will tell you when to take it out. You did such a wonderful job today!"

Steven climbs down to get another toy and then goes out to tell his mother about his adventure.

Appendix C

HOW TO GIVE A PAINLESS INJECTION TO A CHILD

1. Dry the mucosa at the injection site by wiping away all mucous and saliva with a 2x2.

2. Apply topical anesthetic gel and cover with another 2x2 or cotton roll to keep it from being licked off or diluted by saliva.

3. Apply a 50/50 mixture of nitrous oxide and oxygen for a period of 90 seconds through a nosepiece large enough to cover both nose and mouth with no leaks. Note: If the bag is not moving, there is a leak.

4. Stop the flow, remove the nosepiece, and with no delay, gently inject approximately 1/4 cartridge of citanest plain 4% (no vaso-constrictor) using a 30–gauge extra-short needle.

5. Wait 3–5 minutes and re-inject in the exact same site using any needle and any anesthetic. Use the same 90–second nitrous oxide technique for the second injection. There is no need for an oxygen flush with the 90–second technique.

6. Septocaine disperses well through the mandibular bone of young children. Consider infiltration for lower primary molars. It is 4%, so dosage is important.

7. Try the "drip" technique:

- While the child is watching, place a cartridge of citanist plain in a syringe.

- Then screw on a 30–gauge extra-short needle and uncover it.

- Tell the child they do not have to get a shot but instead you will be using the drip method. Demonstrate on your own ungloved finger how it works. Holding the tip of the needle about ½ inch from your fingertip, allow one drop of anesthetic to free fall onto your skin. Wipe it off immediately, explaining to the child that you are doing this "so your finger won't go to sleep."

- Then say, "Now it is your turn. Watch how easy it is." Drip a drop on their finger and wipe it off.

- Then apply the topical to the dry mucosa, start the nitrous, and give a painless two-step injection, as described above. Deceptive? Maybe. Effective? Very.

A rubber dam is best, but if you don't use force and don't cause pain, the child's behavior will be good and you then may not need the dam as a behavior management tool, especially if you are using a glass ionomer filling material, which is not as sensitive to moisture contamination.

Note: If you think that you won't be able to do a perfect job, tell the parent that the restoration many need replacement in a year or two but that this is a small price to pay for their child having a good memory of the dentist. In my experience, the parents never protest when it is explained in advance.

APPENDIX D

OPTIONS FOR VERY YOUNG CHILDREN

PARENT: PLEASE CIRCLE PREFERENCE AND SIGN BELOW.

1. Restore all decayed teeth at one time under general anesthesia.

For safety, this is done in the hospital with an anesthesiologist. This option is the least time-consuming, but it can be expensive even with insurance. The dental work portion, which must be prepaid, is in addition to the hospital and anesthesia fees.

2. Remove the decayed teeth.

This is also done under general anesthesia but by an oral surgeon. The costs are typically less than hospital restorations. Space maintainers will needed later.

3. Arrest the spreading of decay and delay repairs.

This cost-saving option requires the most parental diligence because of the necessity of dietary changes, home fluoride treatments after eating, and brief dental visits every two months.

Parent _____   Date _____

Parent _____   Date _____

Appendix E

HOW TO ARREST EXISTING DECAY

If your young child has small cavities, there are three things that you can do to arrest the decay and delay repairs until your child is old enough to tolerate standard fillings. However, all three actions must be taken consistently to arrest the decay.

1. APPLY FLUORIDE

For decay-prone children, fluoride supplementation from drinking water or pills plus brushing twice a day is not enough. In addition, your child needs extra fluoride from toothpaste. Place a small amount of toothpaste on your child's front teeth or tongue with your finger after each meal and snack consumed at home. The excess is then spit into a tissue. Children too young to spit should have a rice-sized speck of toothpaste at least four times a day. The fluoride in toothpaste may do more to prevent and heal cavities than the actual cleaning action of a toothbrush.

Keep the toothpaste and tissues on the kitchen counter as a visual reminder. No water, no brush, no mess. It's easy, fast, and effective, but it must be done at least four times a day.

2. Reduce consumption of sweets.

For most families, total elimination of sweets is unrealistic and may lead to a craving. How often they are eaten is a bigger issue than how much. It's better for the teeth if sweets are eaten or drunk just once a day with meals and all at one time rather than snacking on them throughout the day. Birch sugar (xylitol) is an excellent sugar substitute because it's safe, tastes good, and reduces cavities. Go to www. sprydental.com

On holidays and birthdays, when there may be more sweets around than usual, after children have eaten their fill, the "sweets fairy" can come at midnight, take what is left, and leave a small or prize or coin.

Note: Apple juice (whether full-strength or diluted), granola, and dried fruit have a similar effect on teeth as candy.

3. Schedule surface applications every two months.

There are decay-inhibiting medications that can be applied to the teeth every two months by the dentist. These are an essential part of arresting decay. They only work well when the recommendations for home fluoride application and sweets reduction are also followed.

Note: You can measure your success by noting the color of the decay. As it becomes arrested and inactive, it gets darker. Completely arrested decay is almost black. As soon as your child is able to tolerate conventional dental treatment in the office, the repairs should be done.

BIBLIOGRAPHY

Adair SM, *et al.* Survey of behavior management teaching in pediatric dentistry advanced education programs. *Pediatric Dentistry* 2004;26(2):151-158.

——Survey of members of American Academy of Pediatric Dentists on their use of behavior management techniques. *Pediatric Dentistry* 2004;26(2):159-166.

Addelston KK. Child patient training. *CDS Rev* 1959;38:7-11.

Adelson R, Goldfried M. Modeling and the fearful child patient. *J Dent Child* 1970;37:476-488.

Anusavice KJ. Treatment regimens in preventive and restorative dentistry. *JADA* 1995;126:727-743.

Bailey PM, Talbot A, Taylor P. A comparison of maternal anxiety levels manifested in the child dental patient. *J Dent Child* 1973;40:277-284.

Berggren U, Meynert G. Dental fear and avoidance: Causes, symptoms, and consequences. *JADA* 1984; 109(2):247-251.

Blinkhorn AS, Kay EJ, Atkinson JM, Millar K. Advice for the dental team on coping with the nervous child. *Dent Update* 1990;17:415-419.

Chambers DW. Managing the anxieties of young dental patients. *J Dent Child* 1970;37:263-274.

Chu CH, Lo ECM, Lin HC. Effectiveness of silver diamine fluoride and sodium fluoride varnish in arresting dentin caries in Chinese pre-school children. *J Dent Res* 2002;81(11):767-770.

Clarke JH. Anxious patient management: A practical approach. *Membership Matters.* Newsletter of the Oregon Dental Association. 1996 Jan;1(9).
Toothaches and death. *J Hist Dent* 1999 Mar;47(1):11-13.

Corah NL. Dental anxiety: Assessment, reduction, and increasing patient satisfaction. *Dentistry* 1990;10:5-9, 23-25.

Effect of perceived control on stress reduction in pedodontic patients. *J Dent Res* 1973;52:1261-1264.

Edelstein, BL. The medical management of dental caries. *JADA* 1994;125:31-39.

Frigoletto R.L. Update: Simplified treatment of Baby-Bottle Syndrome. *J Dent Child* 1982;49:374-376.

Gatchel RJ. Impact of a videotaped dental fear reduction program on people who avoid dental treatment. *JADA* 1986;112:218-221.

—. Managing anxiety and pain during dental treatment. *JADA* 1992;123:37-41.

Greenbaum P, Melamed B. Pre-treatment modeling: A technique for reducing children's fear in the dental operatory. *Dent Clin North Am* 1988;32:693-704.

Irish LE, Ginsburg GM, Clarke JH. Basic dental anxiety. *Gen Dentistry* 1994 May-June;42(3):252-255.

Kleinknecht R, Klepac R, Alexander L. Origins and characteristics of fear of dentistry. *JADA* 1973;86:842-848.

Levitas TC. HOME: Hand-over-mouth exercise. *J Dent Child* 1974;41:178-182.

Logan HL, Baron R, Keeley K, Law A, Stein S. Desired control and felt control as mediators of stress in a dental setting. *Health Psychol* 1991;10:352-359.

Machen J, Johnson R. Desensitization, model learning and the dental behavior of children. *J Dent Res* 1974;53:83-86.

McDonald RB. *Dentistry for the Child and Adolescent.* St. Louis: C.V. Mosby Co.,1974: 36.

Meechan RJ, Professor Emeritus, Pediatric Medicine, Oregon Health Sciences University, Portland. Personal communication. 1992.

Melamed B, Weinstein D, Hawes R, Kartin M. Reduction of fear-related dental management problems with use of filmed modeling. *JADA* 1975;90:822-826.

Milgrom P, Fiset L, Melnick S, Weinstein P. The prevalence and practice management consequences of dental fear in a major U.S. city. *JADA* 1988;116:641-647.

Milgrom P, Vignehsa H, Weinstein P. Adolescent dental fear and control: Prevalence and theoretical implications. *Behav Res Ther* 1992;30:367-373.

Milgram P, Weinstein P. Early Childhood Caries: A Team Approach to Prevention and Treatment. Seattle, WA: University of Washington, Department of Continuing Education, 1999: 66-67.

Moline D. Undoing iatrogenic odontophobia. *Gen Dent* 1991;39:273-276.

Moore R, Brodsgaard I, Birn H. Manifestations, acquisition and diagnostic categories of dental fear in a self-referred population. *Behavior Res Ther* 1991;29(1):51-60.

Olsen NH. The first appointment: A mutual evaluation session. *J Dent Child* 1965;32:208-211.

Pawlicki RE. Psychological/behavioral techniques in managing pain and anxiety in the dental patient. *Anesth Prog* 1991;38:120-127.

Perlmuter L, Monty R. The importance of perceived control: Fact or fantasy. *Am Scientist* 1977;65:759-764.

Pike AR. Prevention of anxiety during the first dental visit of a three-year-old child. *General Dentistry* 1995;43:448-451.

Rouleau J, Ladouceur R, Dufour L. Pre-exposure to the first dental treatment. *J Dent Res* 1981;60:30-34.

Seyrek S, Corah N, Pace L. Comparison of three distraction techniques in reducing stress in dental patients. *JADA* 1984;108:327-329.

Sigelman CK, Shaffer DR. *Lifespan Human Development.* Grove, CA: Brooks/Cole Pacific Publishing, 1991; 410.

Sokol D, Sokol S, Sokol C. A review of non-intrusive therapies used to deal with anxiety and pain in the dental office. *JADA* 1985;110:217-222.

Strupp WC. *A Clinical Technique to Give a Painless Injection.* Monograph. Clearwater, FL: Predictable Dentistry Seminars, 1994.

Thompson SC. Will it hurt less if I can control it? *Psychol Bull* 1981;90:89-101.

Wei SH. *Pediatric Dentistry: Total Patient Care.* Philadelphia, PA: Lea & Febiger, 1988; 153.

Weinstein P, Nathan J. The challenge of fearful and phobic children. *Dent Clin North Am* 1988;32:667-692.

Young M. Overcoming pediatric panic. *Dent Econ* 1991;81:45-48.

About the Author

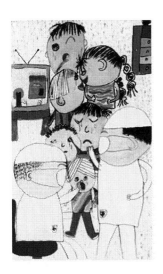 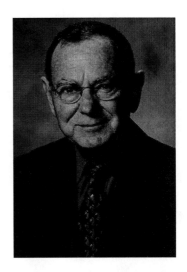

Allan R. Pike, DDS, MS, has had a full-time private practice in pediatric dentistry for 38 years. Over that time, he has delivered scores of presentations on new approaches to behavior management to dentists and dental students in the Pacific Northwest. Dr. Pike is helping to drive a growing concern about the lasting effects on children when they are treated with traditional methods of control in the dental office.

Contact Dr. Pike at www.doctorpike.com or
dentistryforchildren@yahoo.com.

978-0-595-39184-4
0-595-39184-2

2487884

Made in the USA